750

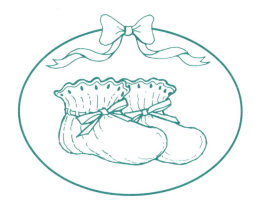

The First Twelve Months of Life

Companion

A Personal Record of
Your Baby's Early Development

The Princeton Center for Infancy and Early Childhood
Theresa Caplan, general editor

Illustrated and designed by Lisa Amoroso

A PERIGEE BOOK

Perigee Books
are published by
The Putnam Publishing Group
200 Madison Avenue
New York, NY 10016

ISBN 0-399-51736-7
Front cover photograph © Photo Media Ltd./H. Armstrong Roberts
Printed in the United States of America
2 3 4 5 6 7 8 9 10

This book is printed on acid-free paper.
∞

ACKNOWLEDGMENTS

Although out of print, there was merit in *Growing-Up Years: Your Child's Record-Keeping Book* which was published by Anchor Press/Doubleday in 1978. Thus, when asked to prepare a less extensive record-keeping book for the first twelve months of life, we deemed it a viable project and responded with alacrity. The late Frank Caplan, founder and general manager of The Princeton Center for Infancy and Early Childhood, would have welcomed this new undertaking.

Of course, we value the contributions of all concerned professionals and practitioners in the fields of early childhood growth and development and parenting education.

We appreciate the efforts of Mrs. Virginia Marino Miller, assistant editor at Perigee Books, on behalf of this work, as well as Mrs. Angela Cox, of Marie Brown Associates, for introducing the author to the publisher.

Wholeheartedly, we thank our good friend Mrs. Dorothy J. Naylor for her practical input and great patience in helping to ready our manuscript for delivery to the publisher.

Theresa Caplan, general editor and author
The Princeton Center for Infancy
and Early Childhood
July 1991

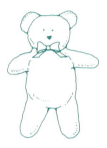

CONTENTS

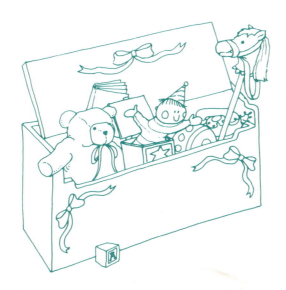

INTRODUCTION

This record-keeping book is intended for prospective or new parents who have purchased or were gifted with *The First Twelve Months of Life: Your Baby's Growth Month by Month.*

Of course, it can be used by all parents who would like an organized format for recording important and interesting data on their baby's earliest months of life.

Birth is the best time to begin this lifetime record. Through the process of joyfully tracking your baby's progress, you will create a unique product: a personal, detailed, and informative record of your baby. This alone is useful, but we at The Princeton Center for Infancy and Early Childhood attach equal value to the process itself. Keeping records will increase your confidence in being able to read your infant's signals and, at the same time, sensitize you to the real expert on infant growth and development—your baby!

We want to emphasize that babies grow and develop at their own, very personal rates and styles. Do not expect that your baby will conform to any specific schedule of development.

The Princeton Center for Infancy and Early Childhood is deeply committed to the principle that mothers and fathers need to assume responsibility jointly for their child and to learn to recognize the individuality of every baby. We have used the word *parents* unless referring specifically to the mother or the father. For lack of a universal pronoun, we have used *he* and *she* randomly with regard to male and female babies.

We have tried to make it easier for you to keep a running account of your baby's upgrowth since slips of paper usually get lost. Try to jot down your answers to the queries without feeling unduly pressured. You, your child when grown, and other close family members will surely enjoy reminiscing about this precise scenario of your precious baby's first twelve months of life.

Above all, enjoy your baby! Although parenting will always be demanding, there is no other role in life that is as challenging or as deeply rewarding.

*This book is lovingly dedicated to
Frank Caplan,
a champion of the best interests
of infants and toddlers and
their concerned parents everywhere.*

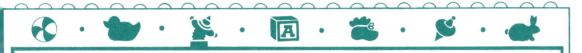

Part One

VITAL
STATISTICS
AND
RECORDS

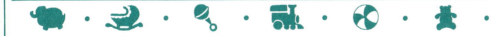

PREGNANCY RECORD

Since many prenatal influences affect the fetus, this record is important to mother and baby and might be useful to the pediatrician.

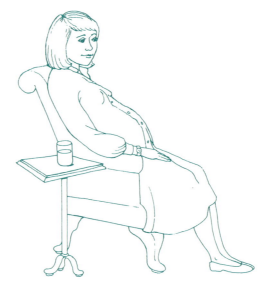

Medication During Pregnancy	Dates	Amount	What Stage of Pregnancy
vitamins	_____	_____	_____
iron	_____	_____	_____
aspirin	_____	_____	_____
laxatives	_____	_____	_____
antihistamines	_____	_____	_____
nasal decongestants	_____	_____	_____
others:	_____	_____	_____
	_____	_____	_____
	_____	_____	_____

chest X ray   _____   _____   _____

other X rays   _____   _____   _____

_____   _____   _____

First sign of life: Date _____   Describe _____

_____

_____

Describe baby's   _____

   reactions to   _____

   external influences,   _____

   eg., sound   _____

Baby's most active time   _____

   of day   _____

Length of Pregnancy

(circle appropriate figures)

28 wks or less	29 to 32 wks	33 to 36 wks	full term (40 wks)	1 to 2 wks past maturity	3 wks or more past maturity

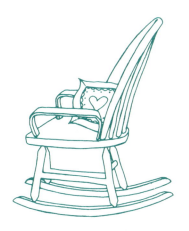

RECORD OF BIRTH

Full name _____

Named for _____

Birth date_____at_____o'clock A.M./P.M.

Place _____
Home or Hospital Name

Address _____
Street   *City*   *State*   *Zip*

Sex____Weight at birth_____Length *(inches)* _____

Skin color_____Eye color_____Hair color _____

Blood type_____Birth order *(1st, 2nd child)* _____

Full-term baby_____Premature birth _____

Personal physician _____
Name   *Address*

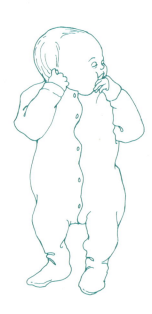

Method of Delivery

Vaginal_____Forceps_____Caesarean section _____

Type of anesthesia used *(if any)* _____

_____

_____

Total time on delivery table _____

Attending doctor's name _____

Address _____

Phone number _____

Attending midwife's name _____

Address _____

Phone number _____

Nurses _____

_____

Father present at birth _____

Baby "roomed-in" _____

Circumcision _____

Other pertinent data *(describe prenatal courses taken, number of sessions, whether father attended)* _____

_____

_____

_____

_____

Left hospital on _____

Feeding: Breast_____Other _____

Formula *(if any)* _____

Any religious ceremony _____

_____

_____

Godfather_____Godmother _____

RECORD OF ADOPTION

The earliest months of the life of every infant are vital to his or her physical well-being, emotional security, and the establishment of social attachments. Therefore, adoptive parents should begin caring for their baby as early as possible.

Full name _____

Baby's birth date _____

Date of adoption _____ Age at adoption _____

Place of adoption _____

How adopted _____

_____

_____

_____

Sex _____ Weight _____ Height _____

Skin color _____ Eye color _____

Hair color _____ Any distinguishing marks _____

_____

Biological parents' history *(if available)* _____

_____

_____

_____

_____

Prior foster parents *(if any)* _____

_____

_____

_____

Siblings *(if any)* _____

_____

VALUABLE DOCUMENTS

The documents that are created in the earliest months can serve your child's best interests throughout life. A birth certificate, record of immunizations, and early illnesses will be essential for attending school, and later for obtaining passports, inheriting property, and so on.

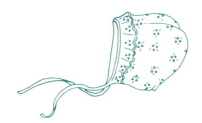

Birth Certificate

Birth Certificate No. _____

Recorded at _____
Place and date

Attach <u>copy</u> of birth certificate here.
If it is too large, ask a copy center for
a one-third reduction. Keep the original
with your important papers.

Immunization Schedule

The American Academy of Pediatrics recommends that children be immunized and given the tuberculin test according to the immunization schedule below. Vaccine schedules and combinations are constantly being improved, so consult your pediatrician for the current timetable. Record the month and year each immunization was completed and any special reactions that occurred.

Baby's Age	Name of Inoculation	Disease to be Resisted	Date Received	Reaction (if any)
2 mos.	DTP Vaccine	Diphtheria, Tetanus, Pertussis (Whooping Cough)	————	————
	Polio Vaccine (first dose)	Polio	————	————
4 mos.	DTP Vaccine (second shot)	Diphtheria, etc. as above	————	————
	Polio Vaccine (second dose)	Polio	————	————
6 mos.	DTP Vaccine completed	Diphtheria, etc. as above	————	————
12 mos.	Tuberculin Test	Tuberculosis	————	————
15 mos.	Measles Vaccine	Red Measles	————	————
	Mumps Vaccine	Mumps	————	————
	Rubella	German Measles	————	————
18 mos.	DTP Booster	Diphtheria, etc. as above	————	————
	Polio Vaccine (completed)	Polio	————	————

Medical History

This record of illnesses, accidents, and X rays (if any) will provide a complete medical history of your growing baby. It will also give a physician access to X rays already taken. This will save you money and, more important, it will avoid the harmful effects of repeating unnecessary X rays.

Illness or Accident	Date	Severity/ Complications/ Treatment	Attending Doctor

YOUR NEWBORN'S IDENTIFICATION MARKS

Any two of the marks below will serve as identification for your baby.

Birthmarks

Give location and diagram to indicate size and shape.

Baby's Palmprints

Baby's Footprints

MEDICAL CHECKUPS

You can use the form below when you take your baby in for monthly checkups. Jot down your questions and the doctor's answers and recommendations. Use a separate sheet for each checkup.

Date of exam _____

Physician _____

Address _____

Baby's age_____Weight_____Height _____

Your questions _____

_____

_____

_____

_____

Doctor's recommendations _____

_____

_____

_____

_____

Your comments _____

_____

_____

_____

_____

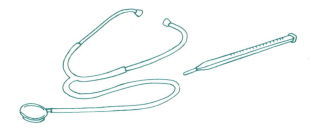

MEMENTOS

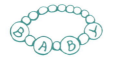 Hospital Bracelet

Announcement of Birth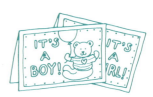

Lock of Baby's Hair

PHOTOGRAPHIC RECORD
OF BIRTH OR ADOPTION

BABY'S FIRST GIFTS

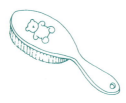 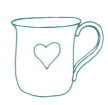 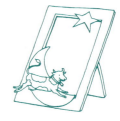

Description   *Donor*

_____

_____

_____

_____

_____

_____

_____

_____

_____

_____

_____

_____

_____

_____

_____

_____

_____

_____

_____

_____

_____

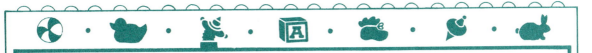

Part Two

YOUR BABY'S DEVELOPMENTAL LANDMARKS

It is important to keep in mind that there is no fixed timetable for a baby's growth and development. Babies eventually pass through the same stages (with rare exceptions). If you have any questions, do talk to your baby's pediatrician.

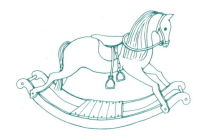

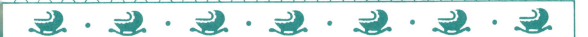

THE FIRST WEEK

Your newborn spends his first week adjusting to his life-sustaining functions and his new environment. It's normal for his heartbeat and breathing to be twice as fast as an adult's. Gradually, his color and skin tone are improving, and his body is filling out.

Reflexes govern your baby's actions (see pages 120–121); twitches, jerky startles, and convulsive movements occur frequently. He usually sleeps from 14 to 18 hours a day. On the average, he is alert and comfortable for only thirty minutes of a 4-hour period. He is very sensitive to pressure and may quiet down when you place your hand on him. Your baby also feels changes in temperature, distinguishes tastes, and responds to light and sounds.

Of course, babies are not physically or psychologically alike at birth, and they have their own unique behavioral styles. The sooner you are able to identify your baby's special temperament—mild-mannered, intense, changeable, and so on—the easier and more enjoyable life will be for you, your baby, and the entire family.

· · · · · · 🍼 · · · · · ·

Weight＿＿＿＿＿Length＿＿＿＿＿Head circumference ＿＿＿＿＿

Does your baby cry a lot?

＿＿＿＿＿＿＿＿＿＿＿＿＿＿＿＿＿＿＿＿＿＿＿＿＿＿＿＿＿＿

＿＿＿＿＿＿＿＿＿＿＿＿＿＿＿＿＿＿＿＿＿＿＿＿＿＿＿＿＿＿

•

Can crooning calm your crying baby?

＿＿＿＿＿＿＿＿＿＿＿＿＿＿＿＿＿＿＿＿＿＿＿＿＿＿＿＿＿＿

＿＿＿＿＿＿＿＿＿＿＿＿＿＿＿＿＿＿＿＿＿＿＿＿＿＿＿＿＿＿

•

When did Baby lose her jaundiced look?

＿＿＿＿＿＿＿＿＿＿＿＿＿＿＿＿＿＿＿＿＿＿＿＿＿＿＿＿＿＿

＿＿＿＿＿＿＿＿＿＿＿＿＿＿＿＿＿＿＿＿＿＿＿＿＿＿＿＿＿＿

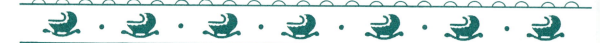

Does Baby wiggle or kick actively?

_____

_____

•

Does Baby fling his arms and legs in all directions?

_____

_____

•

Does Baby make crawling movements when laid flat on her abdomen?

_____

_____

•

Is Baby responding to sudden changes with his whole body?

_____

_____

•

Can your baby move her head from side to side?

_____

_____

•

possibly up and down?

_____

_____

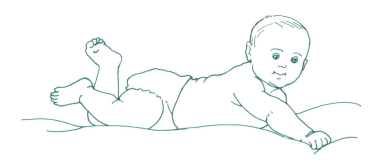

On his abdomen, does Baby lay in a floppy, froglike position

_____

_____

•

or rolled into a ball?

_____

_____

•

Can your baby raise her head from the surface while in the
prone position?

_____

_____

•

Are your baby's hands fisted?

_____

_____

•

Does Baby vocalize actively?

_____

_____

•

Does your baby react to light and dark?

_____

_____

•

Is Baby reacting to loud sounds?

_____

_____

•

Can Baby focus his eyes 8 inches in front of him?

_____

_____

Does your baby respond to sharply contoured or circular shapes?

_____

_____

•

Does your baby quiet down when picked up?

_____

_____

•

or when you apply steady, firm pressure?

_____

_____

•

Is your baby fussy or quiet?

_____

_____

Is Baby alert for only about 30 minutes in a 4-hour period?

_____

_____

•

Does your baby grip an object when his hand encounters it?

_____

_____

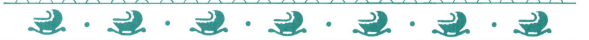

Does Baby stop sucking to look at something?

_____

_____

•

Does your baby search for Mother's nipple?

_____

_____

•

Does Baby move her bowels often and sporadically?

_____

_____

•

Does Baby express disturbance with a frown?

_____

_____

•

with a whimper?

_____

_____

•

or by sucking one or two fingers?

_____

_____

•

How long does your baby sleep?

_____

_____

THE FIRST MONTH

During the first month, you and your family are adjusting to the new member of the household. She in turn continues to adapt to the strange world into which she has been thrust. She spends most of her time sleeping, eating, and crying.

Her muscles are firming up, and she is growing more active—squirming, kicking, or sucking on her fist for long periods of time. When she is alert, really only a small portion of the time she is awake, your baby is gaining better control of her eyes and is able to focus them more quickly and often. She has also begun to make throaty noises, called cooing.

Your baby is slowly settling in. Sleeping and eating patterns are emerging, breathing is becoming more regular, and her jerky startles are reduced to occasional twitches. You need to bear in mind that babies vary in their rate of development, and growth patterns are not necessarily smooth and even. Although children follow the same broad sequences of development, some children even skip one or two stages. For example, some never crawl but instead, they stand up when they "should be" crawling.

Weight_____Length_____Head circumference _____

Does your baby regard your face while you are in his direct line of vision?

_____

_____

•

Has your baby's skin lost its redness?

_____

_____

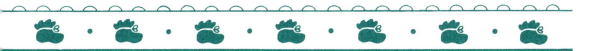

Is your baby's navel completely healed?

_____

_____

•

Are your baby's eyes clear and free of irritation?

_____

_____

•

Record the date your baby first raised her head off your shoulder.

_____

_____

•

Does your baby stop crying when you speak or he sees you?

_____

_____

•

When did your baby's eyes first follow a bright light?

_____

_____

•

Does Baby thrust her arms and legs in play?

_____

_____

•

Does your baby's unsupported head flop backward or forward?

_____

_____

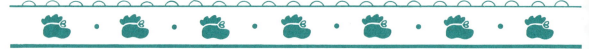

Does your baby roll partway from his side to his back?

_____

_____

•

Can Baby hold her head in line with her back when she is pulled
to sitting position?

_____

_____

•

Is your baby moving around a little bit, enough to squirm to the
corner of the crib?

_____

_____

•

Does Baby keep his hands fisted or slightly open?

_____

_____

•

Does Baby stare at an object, but not yet reach for it?

_____

_____

•

Besides crying, is your baby beginning to make small throaty
sounds?

_____

_____

•

Does your baby prefer patterns to any color?

_____

_____

_____

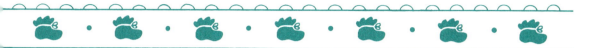

Is your baby alert about 1 out of every 10 hours?

_____

_____

•

Does Baby coordinate her eyes sideways and up and down while regarding a light or an object?

_____

_____

•

Does your baby become excited when he sees a person or a toy?

_____

_____

_____

_____

_____

Is your baby expecting feedings at certain intervals?

_____

_____

•

Does your baby quiet down when held or seeing faces?

_____

_____

•

Does your baby cry deliberately for assistance?

_____

_____

•

Is your baby responding positively to comfort and satisfaction?

_____

_____

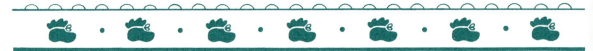

negatively to pain?

_____

_____

•

Does Baby make eye-to-eye contact with Mother, Father, or other constant caretaker?

_____

_____

•

Does your baby root and suck vigorously at breast?

_____

_____

•

suck vigorously on bottle?

_____

_____

•

Is Baby recognizing Mother's and/or Father's voice?

_____

_____

•

How many night feedings does your baby take (2 are average)?

_____

_____

•

how many daytime feedings (5 or 6 are average)?

_____

_____

•

Does your baby move her bowels 3 or 4 times daily?

_____

_____

THE SECOND MONTH

Perhaps the most exciting second-month event is when you see your baby smile. You will notice that he is becoming more active, especially when he's on his back. He is also learning to control his head. His movements are smoother and voluntary grasping is replacing his reflex grasp. He has begun to eat and sleep regularly every day, and even to cry at fairly predictable times. Just as he reacts positively with a smile, he can express his feelings of discomfort and disgust. He also indicates his preferences: for people over objects; for one side of his body over the other while he sleeps.

Babies see well at six weeks, finger and touch from six to twelve weeks, kick with intention at twelve to twenty weeks. As these sensory powers mature, you will notice that your baby is eager to practice his new abilities. He concentrates his full powers to see and to pay attention to all kinds of cues. His mouth functions as an all-purpose sense organ.

Parents or consistent caregivers can enrich the infant's world with sense experiences, using things around the house. However, beware of bombarding your baby with too many sound and sight experiences. An infant also needs quiet time in which to learn and practice. When babies do things over and over again, they are adding information to their memory banks.

· · · · · · 🦆 · · · · · ·

Weight_____Length_____Head circumference _____

Does your baby smile?

_____

_____

·

Is Baby making several different sounds, including cooing?

_____

_____

Does your baby turn her head when she hears a voice?

_____

_____

•

Are Baby's eyes following the movements of persons in the room?

_____

_____

•

Can your baby cycle his arms and legs smoothly?

_____

_____

•

When your baby is on her abdomen, can she keep her head in mid-position?

_____

_____

When he is on his back, can your baby turn his head from side to side easily?

_____

_____

•

When held, does Baby have some control of her neck?

_____

_____

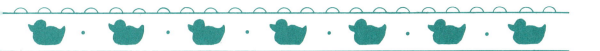

Does her head jerk and bob, but no longer sag forward?

_____

_____

•

Has your baby's grasp become voluntary?

_____

_____

•

Can your baby hold a rattle for a few moments or maybe even longer?

_____

_____

•

Does your baby swipe at nearby objects?

_____

_____

•

Can Baby make a single vowel sound, e.g., *ah, eh, uh?*

_____

_____

•

Does your baby startle at sudden sounds?

_____

_____

•

or respond facially?

_____

_____

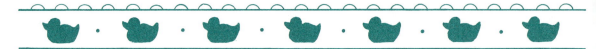

Does your baby stare endlessly at his surroundings?

_____

_____

•

Can Baby focus her eyes on objects at 7 or 8 inches?

_____

_____

•

Has your baby begun to show a preference for his right or left side?

_____

_____

•

Does your baby clearly discriminate among voices?

_____

_____

•

people?

_____

_____

•

tastes?

_____

_____

•

proximity?

_____

_____

•

object size?

_____

_____

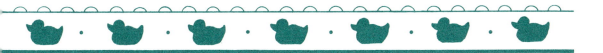

Does Baby show distress?

_____

_____

•

excitement?

_____

_____

•

delight?

_____

_____

Can your baby quiet herself with sucking?

_____

_____

•

Does Baby regard you alertly and directly?

_____

_____

•

Has your baby's body tone improved?

_____

_____

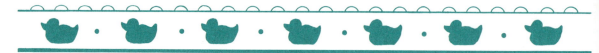

Does your baby have only 1 night feeding?

_____

_____

•

Does Baby move his bowels twice a day close to feedings?

_____

_____

•

Is your baby awake as many as 10 hours a day?

_____

_____

•

Does Baby have 2 to 4 longer sleep periods?

_____

_____

•

Does your baby enjoy her bath?

_____

_____

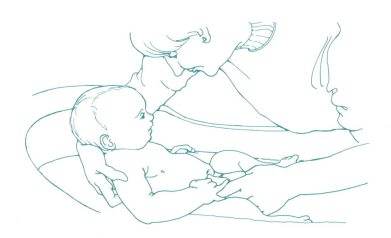

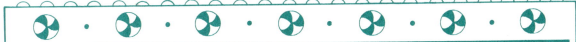

THE THIRD MONTH

Your baby is gradually growing more aware of herself and of the people and things that surround her. You'll see evidence of her memory development as she begins to recognize and differentiate family members. Everyone responds to her cooing (vowel-like, one-syllable sounds) and, especially, her spontaneous, most appealing smiles. She will vocalize when you talk to her, much to your mutual delight.

Indiscriminate crying decreases dramatically by your baby's third-month birthday. Her tonic neck reflex is disappearing. In fact, she is starting to integrate her reflex and voluntary behaviors. For example, her grasping has become voluntary. She has better control of her body and can sit supported with a minimum of head bobbing.

Educators and researchers report that early play life has a profound influence on a baby's motor and sensory development, overall learning, as well as budding self-image. Watch as your baby inititiates play by looking at and playing with her hands and swiping at objects. You can provide your baby with other simple, enjoyable, stimulating play experiences. Games that please both infant and parents can be started when your baby is about three months old.

· · · · · · 🔵 · · · · · ·

Weight_____Length_____Head circumference _____

Does your baby switch from reflex to voluntary body movements?

_____

_____

•

Has your baby's head control improved markedly?

_____

_____

Is your baby's tonic neck reflex disappearing?

_____

_____

•

While on her back, does your baby keep her body straight?

_____

_____

•

Does your baby hold his head firmly when held to your shoulder?

_____

_____

•

Can your baby sit supported with a minimum of head bobbing?

_____

_____

•

Does your baby keep her hands mostly open?

_____

_____

•

Can Baby roll from his back to his side?

_____

_____

•

Is your baby able to raise herself by pushing up on her arms
when on her abdomen?

_____

_____

•

Does Baby play with his fingers?

_____

_____

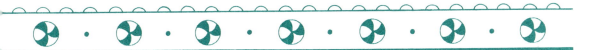

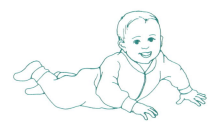

Do your baby's eyes follow a moving object?

_____

_____

•

Can she turn her head freely to follow moving objects or people?

_____

_____

•

Does your baby indicate pleasure by making sounds?

_____

_____

•

Does your baby hold his head erect?

_____

_____

•

Can your baby be pacified by your voice or pleasant sounds?

_____

_____

•

When pulled to stand, does Baby press her feet against the surface and stand briefly?

_____

_____

•

Does your baby coo one-syllable, vowel-like sounds, i.e., *ooh, ah, ae?*

_____

_____

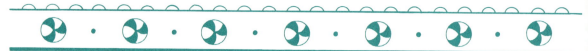

Does your baby definitely respond to your smile and talk by cooing and smiling back?

_____

_____

•

Does Baby listen to voices?

_____

_____

•

Is your baby attentive up to ¾ of an hour at a time?

_____

_____

•

Does your baby respond facially to an object?

_____

_____

•

Can Baby concentrate on a picture or a toy close up or in the distance?

_____

_____

•

Does your baby glance from one object to another?

_____

_____

•

Does Baby regard a dangling object in front of him promptly?

_____

_____

•

swipe at the object with closed fist?

_____

_____

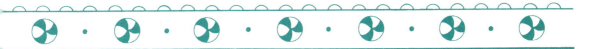

or reach for it with both hands?

_____

_____

•

Is your baby experimenting with changes in proximity by drawing in and extending her arm?

_____

_____

•

Does Baby glance at a rattle in your hand?

_____

_____

•

try to play with the rattle?

_____

_____

•

Is your baby becoming bored with repeated sounds or images?

_____

_____

•

Does your baby calm quickly to concentrate on a face?

_____

_____

•

Has Baby begun to recognize and differentiate family members?

_____

_____

•

Does your baby watch his hands and feet at length?

_____

_____

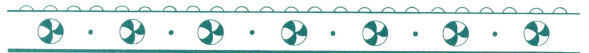

Does Baby stop sucking to listen?

_____

_____

•

Is your baby responding to most kinds of stimulation with her
whole body?

_____

_____

•

Has your baby's swallowing and grasping become voluntary?

_____

_____

•

Is Baby smiling immediately and spontaneously?

_____

_____

•

Has your baby's crying decreased dramatically?

_____

_____

•

Does your baby squeal with frustration?

_____

_____

•

whimper with hunger?

_____

_____

•

smack lips?

_____

_____

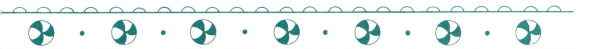

Will Baby stop or start crying according to who holds him?

_____

_____

•

Does your baby try to attract Mother's or Father's attention?

_____

_____

•

Is your baby turning her head to speaking or singing voices?

_____

_____

•

familiar person's sounds?

_____

_____

•

an approaching adult?

_____

_____

•

Does your baby vocalize when talked to?

_____

_____

Is Baby indicating that he remembers feeding time by opening
his mouth expectantly?

_____

_____

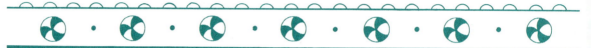

Have you started feeding diluted cereal to your baby (rice, oatmeal, or barley)?

_____

_____

•

Are your baby's patterns of eating clearly established?

_____

_____

•

of being alert?

_____

_____

•

of sleeping?

_____

_____

•

Does Baby have one nightly feeding?

_____

_____

•

Is your baby taking 2 naps; a couple of hours in the morning and a couple in the afternoon?

_____

_____

•

Does your baby sleep about 10 hours a night?

_____

_____

•

Has your baby chosen a favorite position for sleeping?

_____

_____

THE FOURTH MONTH

This month you'll see your baby grow more responsive to his "outside world" and more eager to become a social being. Now he not only smiles freely, but he has added laughing and babbling to his language repertoire.

Your baby can turn his head in all directions whether lying down or seated, and roll from side to side while on his abdomen. The Moro reflex is waning. He has better control of his fingers and uses his hands playfully and purposefully. His vision is almost that of an adult, and he is able to turn his head and eyes in coordination. You can tell that his memory span has increased to five or seven minutes. He may even be able to wait for a feeding, which may now include solid foods—a milestone. (You may spot his two lower front teeth coming in!)

Your four-month-old shows an interest in playthings, and he may prefer one toy. He especially enjoys physical play, games, and socializing. Music continues to have a soothing effect.

· · · · · · 🐰 · · · · · ·

Weight_____Length_____Head circumference _____

Is your baby's Moro reflex beginning to vanish?

_____

_____

•

When on her back, does your baby keep her head in mid-position?

_____

_____

•

Can your baby turn his head in all directions, prone or seated?

_____

_____

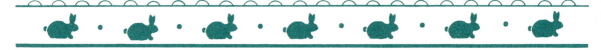

Does your baby hold her head erect and steady for a short time?

_____

_____

•

Is Baby turning his head toward voices?

_____

_____

•

When on her abdomen, does your baby lift her head 90 degrees from surface?

_____

_____

•

on straight arms?

_____

_____

•

or with weight on forearms?

_____

_____

•

When on his back, does your baby crane his neck forward to see his hands catch his feet?

_____

_____

•

When on her abdomen, does your baby rock like an airplane, limbs extended and back arched?

_____

_____

•

When on his abdomen, does your baby roll from side to side?

_____

_____

Is your baby on the verge of rolling over?

_____

_____

•

If pulled to stand, does your baby extend her legs and keep her
body in the same plane from shoulders to feet?

_____

_____

•

Can your baby sit propped up for 10 to 15 minutes with his head
erect and steady and his back firm?

_____

_____

•

Is your baby using her hands with more agility and variety of
movements?

_____

_____

Can your baby hold on to small objects?

_____

_____

•

hold a rattle?

_____

_____

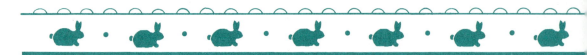

Is there the beginning of coordination between your baby's eyes and his body movements?

_____

_____

•

Does your baby laugh aloud?

_____

_____

•

Has Baby begun babbling (strings of syllable-like vocalizing)?

_____

_____

•

When talked to, does your baby smile, squeal, or coo?

_____

_____

•

Does Baby grin when pleased?

_____

_____

Can your baby imitate several different tones?

_____

_____

•

Has your baby increased her responsive periods to an hour or more at a time?

_____

_____

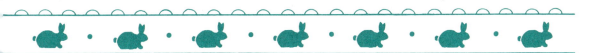

Has your baby become adept at focusing his eyes on brightly colored objects?

_____

_____

•

Is your baby visually exploring her environment?

_____

_____

•

Does Baby follow dangling or moving objects?

_____

_____

•

Does your baby regard a teether or rattle immediately?

_____

_____

•

Can Baby pull an object toward him?

_____

_____

•

Does your baby carry an object to her mouth?

_____

_____

•

Can your baby swipe with one arm and open hand, but often miss?

_____

_____

•

Does Baby stare at the place from which an object drops?

_____

_____

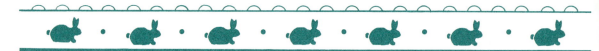

Does your baby know Mother, Father, or other constant caretaker?

_____

_____

•

Has your baby discovered that he can use his fingers separately?

_____

_____

•

Does Baby look down at her hands?

_____

_____

•

clasp his fingers and hands in play?

_____

_____

Does your baby smile and vocalize at her mirror image?

_____

_____

•

Does your baby prefer one toy to another?

_____

_____

•

Can your baby transfer a toy or object from one hand to the other?

_____

_____

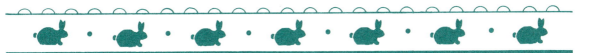

Does Baby vocalize his moods?

_____

_____

•

Does your baby laugh while socializing?

_____

_____

•

Will Baby wail if play is interrupted?

_____

_____

•

Does your baby show anticipation, i.e., excites, breathes heavily?

_____

_____

•

Does your baby attempt to soothe herself?

_____

_____

•

Is your baby quieted by music?

_____

_____

•

Does your baby vocalize to initiate socializing?

_____

_____

•

with coughs?

_____

_____

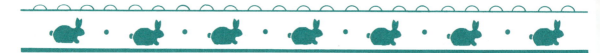

clicking of tongue?

_____

_____

•

Does your baby show interest in playthings?

_____

_____

•

Can your baby wait for a feeding?

_____

_____

•

Does Baby recognize his bottle?

_____

_____

•

purse his mouth for food?

_____

_____

•

Is your baby enjoying new solid foods (puréed fruits and
vegetables) as you offer them?

_____

_____

Does your baby splash and kick in the bath and lift her head?

_____

_____

THE FIFTH MONTH

Your baby has come a long way from her earliest days. She is no longer a limp doll; instead, she is a delightful, automated being full of enchantment and promise. She may locomote by rocking, rolling, and twisting; or on her back, by kicking against a flat surface. She is easily pulled to stand, and can sit supported for about thirty minutes with her back firm.

Crawling and creeping are synonymous terms that describe moving the body close to the ground while using hands and knees in tandem. Babies exhibit some amusing antics before they master this skill. As soon as your baby notices toys, move one slowly a short distance in front of her in order to stimulate the greatest creeping efforts.

She recognizes you as well as the other familiar people and objects in her life. She has learned to smile or vocalize to make social contact, and do not be surprised if she smiles and vocalizes to her mirror image. You may be thrilled to hear a recognizable word, like "dada," as your baby experiments with different sounds.

. . . .

Weight_____Length_____Head circumference _____

Can your baby bring her feet to her mouth and suck on her toes?

_____

_____

•

Does everything automatically go into your baby's mouth?

_____

_____

is there much drooling?

_____

_____

•

When on his back, does your baby lift his head and shoulders?

_____

_____

•

Has your baby rolled over for the first time?

_____

_____

(Never leave your baby unguarded on a bed or other surface from which she or he can fall!)

Has Baby attempted to locomote by rocking, rolling, and twisting?

_____

_____

_____

_____

_____

When supported under the arms, does your baby stand and move body up and down?

_____

_____

•

stamp one foot and then the other?

_____

_____

When seated or pulled to sit, does your baby continuously hold her head steady and erect?

_____

_____

•

Does Baby grasp an object with his thumb and forefinger?

_____

_____

•

Does your baby play with a rattle placed in her hands?

_____

_____

•

Does your baby hold his bottle with 1 hand or 2 hands?

_____

_____

Does your baby reach for a teething ring and grasp it with good aim?

_____

_____

•

Can your baby grab or wave an object with either hand?

_____

_____

•

Does your baby utter vowel-like sounds: *ee, ay, ey, ah, ooh?*

_____

_____

and a few consonant-like sounds: *d, b, l, m?*

_____

_____

•

Does your baby vocalize spontaneously to herself?

_____

_____

•

to toys?

_____

_____

•

Is your baby babbling to gain attention?

_____

_____

•

Does your baby watch people's mouths closely?

_____

_____

•

Does Baby experiment with his own sounds after hearing others'?

_____

_____

•

Does your baby turn her head to human sounds?

_____

_____

•

does she seem to look for the speaker?

_____

_____

Can your baby discriminate his name?

_____

_____

•

Is your baby alert for up to 1½ hours?

_____

_____

•

up to 2 hours?

_____

_____

•

Does your baby look around in new situations?

_____

_____

•

Is Baby turning her head deliberately to a sound?

_____

_____

•

or to follow a disappearing object?

_____

_____

Do your baby's eyes participate in grasping and manipulating an object?

_____

_____

Does your baby raise his hand in the vicinity of an object?

_____

_____

•

glance alternately between hand and object?

_____

_____

•

gradually close gap and grasp object?

_____

_____

•

Is your baby able to reach for an object by moving both hands from her sides to the middle of her body?

_____

_____

•

sometimes with closed fists?

_____

_____

•

Does Baby lean over to look for a fallen object?

_____

_____

Is your baby trying to catch a moving object between his hands?

_____

_____

•

Does your baby want to touch, hold, turn, shake, mouth, and taste objects?

_____

_____

•

Can Baby recognize familiar objects?

_____

_____

•

Is your baby discriminating her parents from others?

_____

_____

•

Does your baby appear to be afraid of strangers, especially women?

_____

_____

(Your baby has begun to recognize the difference between familiar and unfamiliar people.)

Does your baby deliberately imitate sounds and movements?

_____

_____

•

Does your baby show fear?

_____

_____

•

anger?

_____

_____

disgust?

_____

_____

•

Is Baby smiling and vocalizing to his mirror image?

_____

_____

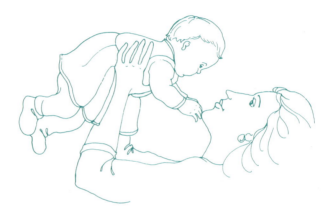

Does your baby raise her arms to be picked up?

_____

_____

•

Is Baby smiling or vocalizing to make social contact?

_____

_____

•

Does your baby make a face in imitation?

_____

_____

•

Has your baby learned to tease?

_____

_____

Does your baby stop crying when talked to?

_____

_____

•

Is Baby frolicsome when played with?

_____

_____

•

Has your baby's interest in breast feeding begun to wane?

_____

_____

•

Does your baby take solid foods well?

_____

_____

•

Has your baby started to drink from a cup?

_____

_____

•

Does your baby wake promptly at dawn?

_____

_____

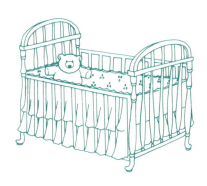

THE SIXTH MONTH

The sixth month is the first month that physical activity is really remarkable, and you'll begin to be aware of your baby's personal style of development. He will probably enjoy clowning around, playing games, and trying out his new physical and social abilities.

Your six-month-old can stand with substantial support, and balance well while sitting with slight support. He may even sit unsupported for up to a half hour. As evidence of his increasing dexterity, he now can pick up a small block directly and deftly, and transfer it from one hand to the other. He may also begin to show an interest in finger-feeding himself.

Since he has more control of the sounds he makes, he vocally expresses pleasure and dissatisfaction, and coos or hums or stops crying upon hearing music. He loves to babble, especially in response to female voices.

Professionals agree that many emotional insecurities develop early if infants are not able to build a feeling of trust and love with one principal caretaker. The period from six to fifteen months is especially critical due to the fears of strangers and abandonment. Therefore, if both Mother and Father are working, great effort should be made to provide a steady, loving substitute caretaker for Baby.

* * * * * * 🚂 * * * * * *

Weight_____Length_____Head circumference _____

Can your baby lift up her chest completely and support herself on her hands and knees?

_____

_____

When on his abdomen, does your baby lift and extend his legs up high?

_____

_____

•

Does your baby turn and twist in all directions?

_____

_____

•

Does Baby get up on her hands and knees in a crouch position and hurtle forward or backward by flinging her limbs out?

_____

_____

•

Can your baby stand with substantial support?

_____

_____

•

Can your baby sit upright with slight support?

_____

_____

•

Can your baby sit unsupported for up to ½ hour?

_____

_____

•

sit in a high chair?

_____

_____

_____

Can your baby grasp objects using all of his fingers?

_____

_____

•

Can your baby rotate her wrist?

_____

_____

•

Can your baby hold two small objects at the same time, one in
each hand?

_____

_____

•

Does your baby move toward objects?

_____

_____

Does your baby play with a spoon, a rattle, or a teething ring?

_____

_____

•

Is your baby varying the volume, pitch, and rate of his
utterances?

_____

_____

•

Is your baby beginning to intersperse vowels with more
consonants—commonly _f, v, th, s, sh, z, sz, m, n?_

_____

_____

Does your baby babble and become active when surrounded by exciting sounds?

_____

_____

•

Is your baby babbling back mostly to female voices?

_____

_____

•

Does Baby vocalize pleasure and displeasure?

_____

_____

•

coo and gurgle with delight?

_____

_____

•

squeal with excitement?

_____

_____

•

grunt or growl to complain?

_____

_____

•

Does your baby giggle or belly laugh?

_____

_____

•

Is Baby reacting to differences in intonations?

_____

_____

Does your baby turn toward sounds?

_____

_____

·

Will your baby coo, hum, or stop crying upon hearing music?

_____

_____

·

Is Baby alert for about 2 hours at a stretch?

_____

_____

·

Is your baby visually alert close to 50% of daylight hours?

_____

_____

·

Does your baby reach persistently and quickly for anything she sees?

_____

_____

·

Can Baby pick up a small block directly and deftly?

_____

_____

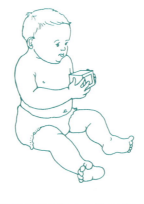

Does your baby like to look at objects upside down to create changes in perspective?

_____

_____

•

Is your baby inspecting objects at length?

_____

_____

•

Does your baby object when he loses his grip on a toy?

_____

_____

•

or is left alone?

_____

_____

(Your baby is becoming increasingly interested in the world around him.)

Is your baby more sociable, i.e., will she look up from what she is doing when people enter the room?

_____

_____

•

Does your baby show an interest in containers?

_____

_____

•

lift inverted containers?

_____

_____

Does your baby differentiate self from mirror image?

_____

_____

•

Is Baby aware of separate parts of himself?

_____

_____

•

Does your baby recognize differences between members of
household and strangers?

_____

_____

•

do strangers disturb your baby?

_____

_____

•

Is your baby smiling at unfamiliar children?

_____

_____

•

reaching out to pat them?

_____

_____

•

Does your baby call you for help?

_____

_____

•

When on her back, will Baby grasp her foot in play?

_____

_____

Does your baby enjoy playing peekaboo?

_____

_____

•

Is your baby showing an interest in finger-feeding himself?

_____

_____

Has your baby developed definite taste preferences?

_____

_____

•

Does Baby want to manipulate her bottle?

_____

_____

•

Has your baby started to manipulate his cup?

_____

_____

•

Does Baby sleep about half of a 24-hour period?

_____

_____

•

Is your baby sleeping through the night?

_____

_____

THE SEVENTH MONTH

Along with her advancing motor abilities, your baby continues to explore and to compare herself to her world and the people in it. Her ability to creep continues to improve, and now she can count on going forward all the time. She is beginning to experiment with standing. Her thumb apposition is complete, and she can hold two objects, one in each hand, simultaneously. She is also becoming aware of the size differences of objects.

You may be surprised when your baby resists pressure to do something she does not wish to do. Do not fight this expression of burgeoning independence; instead, direct her to more positive behavior. You'll also notice she is developing a sense of humor.

Your baby may say "dada" and/or "mama" at this time. Stages of language acquisition are universal, but be aware that each baby goes through these stages in her own way, at her own rate. Some linguists and psychologists believe that speech is tied to a child's motor development and unfolds naturally. A few claim that it results from interaction with parents. Nonetheless, babies who have parents who talk to them seem to talk more.

· · · · · · 🪀 · · · · · ·

Weight_____Height_____Head circumference _____

Does your baby balance her head well?

_____

_____

•

Is Baby trying to poke at available objects?

_____

_____

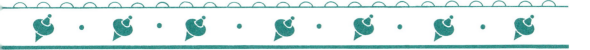

Can your baby creep with an object in one hand?

_____

_____

•

or objects in both hands?

_____

_____

Does Baby go forward by sitting and bouncing on his buttocks?

_____

_____

•

by sitting on the side of his flexed leg and propelling himself
with corresponding hand and opposite leg?

_____

_____

•

or by standing, lunging, and grabbing at furniture?

_____

_____

•

Does your baby pull herself to stand?

_____

_____

•

When supported under his arms, does your baby stand and bear
his weight?

_____

_____

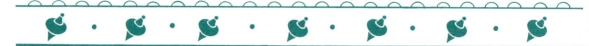

step in place?

_____

_____

•

look at his feet?

_____

_____

•

Does your baby get herself to sit by pushing up with her arms
from her sides?

_____

_____

•

or by getting into crawl position and sticking legs out in front?

_____

_____

•

Can your baby use his thumb and other fingers to grasp a block?

_____

_____

•

Is your baby banging 2 objects together?

_____

_____

•

Does your baby have well-defined syllables, usually 4 or more,
that sound like *ma, mu, da, di, ba?*

_____

_____

•

Is your baby trying to imitate sounds or sound sequences?

_____

_____

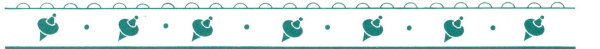

Can your baby say "dada" and/or "mama"?

_____

_____

•

Does your baby listen to her own vocalizations?

_____

_____

•

and those of others?

_____

_____

•

Is your baby's attention span more concentrated?

_____

_____

•

Can your baby reach for and grasp a small toy with one hand?

_____

_____

Does Baby distinguish near and far objects and space?

_____

_____

•

Is your baby playing vigorously with noisemaking toys (i.e., a rattle, bell block, etc.)?

_____

_____

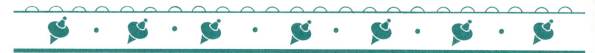

Is Baby responding with expectation to the repetition of an event or signal?

_____

_____

•

Has your baby started to imitate an act?

_____

_____

•

Does your baby visually associate his acts and similar acts of another person?

_____

_____

•

Does your baby reach for and pat her mirror image?

_____

_____

Is your baby exploring his body with his mouth and hands?

_____

_____

•

Does your baby show signs of humor?

_____

_____

•

Has your baby indicated a desire to be included in social interactions?

_____

_____

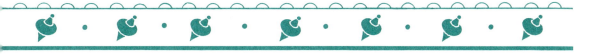

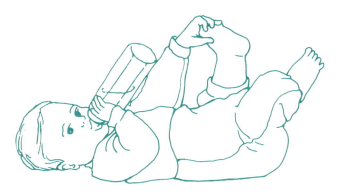

Does your baby resist pressure to do something she doesn't want
to do?

_____

_____

•

Does Baby chew his fingers or suck his thumb?

_____

_____

•

Does your baby play with her toys?

_____

_____

•

Is your baby finger-feeding himself?

_____

_____

•

Is your baby holding and manipulating a spoon or cup in play?

_____

_____

•

Does your baby stay dry for 1 or 2 hours at a time?

_____

_____

THE EIGHTH MONTH

Now that he has mastered crawling, your eight-month-old is learning to stand. One way he does this is by pulling himself up on furniture, but he will still need help to get down from standing. In addition, he can sit alone for several minutes. He has a fine pincer grasp and tries to pick up everything in sight.

Your baby is beginning to recognize some familiar words, and he may now use "Dada" and/or "Mama" as specific names, to the great joy of his parents. He shouts for attention, and may even push away something he does not want. He especially dislikes confinement and lets you know this in no uncertain terms. He has a definite personality.

Due to increasing mobility in this and the upcoming months, your baby is open to a wide variety of stimulating experiences. You should be alert to his reactions to them. Now is a good time to have your baby's hearing checked; no age is too young for the detection of any problems.

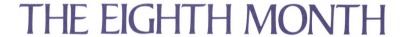

Weight＿＿＿＿＿Height＿＿＿＿＿Head circumference ＿＿＿＿＿

Can your baby change from a lying to a sitting position without help?

＿＿＿＿＿＿＿＿＿＿＿＿＿＿＿＿＿＿＿＿＿＿＿＿＿＿＿＿＿＿＿＿＿

＿＿＿＿＿＿＿＿＿＿＿＿＿＿＿＿＿＿＿＿＿＿＿＿＿＿＿＿＿＿＿＿＿

•

Does your baby crawl?

＿＿＿＿＿＿＿＿＿＿＿＿＿＿＿＿＿＿＿＿＿＿＿＿＿＿＿＿＿＿＿＿＿

＿＿＿＿＿＿＿＿＿＿＿＿＿＿＿＿＿＿＿＿＿＿＿＿＿＿＿＿＿＿＿＿＿

•

with one hand full?

＿＿＿＿＿＿＿＿＿＿＿＿＿＿＿＿＿＿＿＿＿＿＿＿＿＿＿＿＿＿＿＿＿

＿＿＿＿＿＿＿＿＿＿＿＿＿＿＿＿＿＿＿＿＿＿＿＿＿＿＿＿＿＿＿＿＿

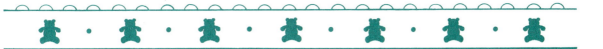

Does your baby stand leaning against something, hands free?

_____

_____

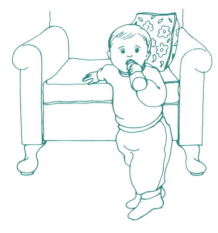

Is your baby pulling on furniture to stand?

_____

_____

•

Does your baby need help to get down from standing?

_____

_____

•

Can your baby stand by holding onto someone's hand?

_____

_____

•

Held standing, does your baby put one foot in front of the other?

_____

_____

•

Does your baby sit and bounce on his buttocks?

_____

_____

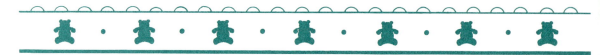

Can your baby's thumb, first, and second fingers grasp a block?

_____

_____

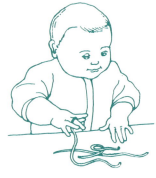

Does your baby use thumb and forefinger in a pincer grasp?

_____

_____

•

can she pick up string?

_____

_____

•

Does your baby reach for objects with fingers overextended?

_____

_____

•

Is your baby babbling with a variety of sounds and inflections?

_____

_____

•

spontaneously?

_____

_____

•

for fun?

_____

_____

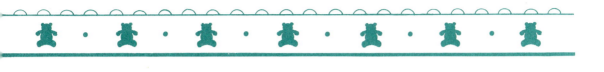

still primarily for self?

_____

_____

•

Does your baby shout?

_____

_____

•

Can Baby mimic your mouth and jaw movements?

_____

_____

•

Is your baby making two-syllable utterances?

_____

_____

•

Does your baby usually respond (turn head and torso) to familiar
nearby sounds?

_____

_____

•

to his or her name?

_____

_____

•

to the telephone?

_____

_____

•

to the vacuum cleaner?

_____

_____

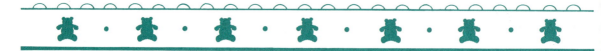

to the alarm clock?

_____

_____

•

Does your baby appear to recognize some familiar words?

_____

_____

•

Is your baby examining objects as external, three-dimensional realities?

_____

_____

•

Does your baby recall a past event as well as a past action of his own?

_____

_____

•

Does your baby anticipate events independent of her own behavior?

_____

_____

•

Is your baby beginning to show memory of timing?

_____

_____

•

Does Baby have a mental model of the human face?

_____

_____

•

Does your baby try to solve simple problems, i.e., kicking at hanging toy to try to get it?

_____

_____

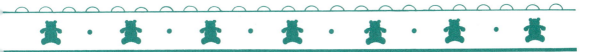

ringing bell purposely?

_____

_____

•

pulling string to secure attached toy?

_____

_____

•

Does your baby pat, smile at, and try to kiss mirror image?

_____

_____

•

Is Baby protesting being separated from Mother?

_____

_____

•

Does your baby quiet down when Mother talks to him?

_____

_____

•

Does your baby push away something she does not want?

_____

_____

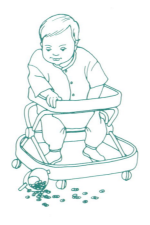

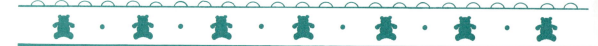

Is Baby rejecting confinement?

_____

_____

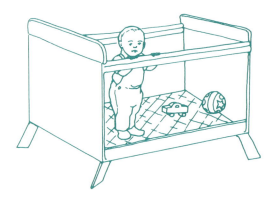

Does your baby know how to use parents to get things for him?

_____

_____

•

Is Baby reaching persistently for toys beyond her reach?

_____

_____

•

Does your baby sustain interest in play?

_____

_____

•

Is Baby still enjoying the "I throw it down—you pick it up" game?

_____

_____

•

Does your baby have trouble sleeping?

_____

_____

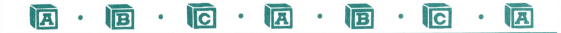

THE NINTH MONTH

During the ninth month, your baby is polishing both her physical skills, such as crawling and standing, and her mental skills. For instance, she may get herself to stand without pulling up on furniture, and get down from standing smoothly. She may side-step or "cruise" along furniture, and she sits effortlessly in a chair. Also, you may notice that your baby exhibits an important mental skill: the ability to attend to and use several ideas at once.

Your baby's language skills are improving, and she can imitate coughs, tongue clicks, and hisses. She may be able to carry out simple commands, and anticipate a reward for successfully doing so; for example, "Good baby!" and a hug or a kiss.

You have become increasingly adept at reading your infant's signs of comfort as well as distress. Positive patterns of attachment between you have been established during the past several months. Your ongoing nurturing and love will instill the trust and courage your child will thrive on for the rest of her life.

· · · · · · 🅰 · · · · · ·

Weight_____Height_____Head circumference _____

Can your baby turn around?

_____

_____

·

Can your baby crawl up stairs?

_____

_____

·

Does your baby stand erect briefly with hand held?

_____

_____

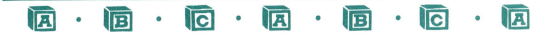

Is your baby actively creeping?

_____

_____

•

Can your baby sit down from standing?

_____

_____

•

Does your baby use his index finger to point, poke into holes, etc.?

_____

_____

Can your baby build a tower of two blocks?

_____

_____

•

Can your baby stand alone briefly?

_____

_____

•

Can your baby stand without pulling up on furniture?

_____

_____

•

Does your baby side-step or "cruise" along furniture?

_____

_____

Can your baby sit steadily and indefinitely alone?

_____

_____

•

Have your baby's intonation patterns become distinct?

_____

_____

•

Does your baby indicate emotions by vocalizing?

_____

_____

•

Is Baby imitating coughs, tongue clicks, and hisses?

_____

_____

•

Does your baby say a syllable or a larger sequence repeatedly?

_____

_____

•

Is your baby listening to conversations?

_____

_____

•

singing tones?

_____

_____

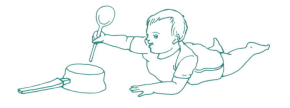

Does your baby understand and respond to 1 or 2 words other than her name, i.e., "no"?

_____

_____

•

Is your baby afraid of heights? (This means that he is aware of vertical space.)

_____

_____

•

Does Baby approach a small object with finger and thumb?

_____

_____

•

a large object with both hands?

_____

_____

•

Does your baby change dimensions of objects by partially covering her eyes or looking upside down?

_____

_____

•

Is your baby dropping 1 of 2 blocks to get a third?

_____

_____

•

Has your baby begun to show a quality of persistence?

_____

_____

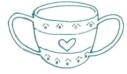

Does your baby recognize Mother and himself in mirror?

_____

_____

•

Does your baby anticipate Mother coming for feeding?

_____

_____

•

Does your baby perform for a home audience?

_____

_____

•

Does your baby repeat an act if applauded?

_____

_____

Is your baby sensitive to other children?

_____

_____

•

will she cry if they cry?

_____

_____

•

Does your baby show an interest in other people's play?

_____

_____

Is your baby initiating play?

_____

_____

•

Does your baby play Pat-a-cake?

_____

_____

•

So-big?

_____

_____

•

Bye-bye?

_____

_____

•

ball games?

_____

_____

•

Is your baby choosing a toy deliberately?

_____

_____

•

Can your baby feed himself a cracker?

_____

_____

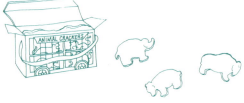

Does your baby hold her bottle?

_____

_____

•

Can your baby drink from a cup?

_____

_____

•

use the cup handle?

_____

_____

•

Does your baby enjoy or fear his bath?

_____

_____

•

Is Baby taking a daytime nap of 1 to 2½ hours?

_____

_____

•

Do you put your baby to bed at the same time every night?

_____

_____

•

Is your baby waking up during the night?

_____

_____

•

Does your baby usually sleep from 12 to 13 hours every night?

_____

_____

93

THE TENTH MONTH

Your baby continues to reinforce his old skills; any new skills he learns will probably be manual. Three major human skills that must be achieved during the early years of life are (1) standing erect and walking; (2) handling simple tools; and (3) organized speech. Once developed, they enable the child to do incredibly inventive and complex things. The manner in which infants achieve these basic skills reflects fundamental principles involved in the growth process. They cannot be considered as either innate or learned; instead, they are a wonderful blend of both. One easy way to see these connections is to support your baby in an upright position from time to time until he gains enough control to stand and move forward on his own two feet.

Your ten-month-old is developing his sense of identity about himself and what belongs to him. He shows moods, looks hurt, sad, happy, uncomfortable, angry, and so on. He can point to his body parts and enjoys playing that game. He is more sensitive toward other children, and shows tenderness toward his stuffed animals or dolls. He helps dress himself and can feed himself whole meals. You are justifiably proud of his accomplishments.

Weight_____Height_____Head circumference _____

Does your baby crawl on straightened limbs?

_____
_____

Can your baby stand with little support?

_____
_____

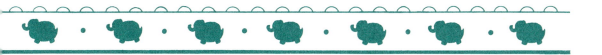

Does your baby walk when you hold
both of his hands?

_____
_____
_____
_____

•

Does your baby climb up and down from chairs?

_____
_____

•

Can your baby sit down smoothly from standing?

_____
_____

•

Does your baby get onto her abdomen from a sitting position?

_____
_____

•

Can Baby carry 2 small objects in one hand?

_____
_____

•

Does Baby enjoy dangling an object from a string?

_____
_____

•

Does your baby differentiate the use of his hands, i.e., holding
with one and maneuvering with the other?

_____
_____

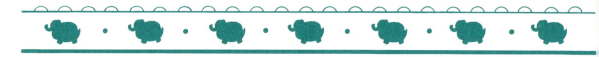

Has your baby learned some words and appropriate gestures,
i.e., says *No* and shakes head?

_____

_____

•

says *Bye-bye* and waves?

_____

_____

•

Has your baby begun to imitate definite intelligible sounds?

_____

_____

•

Does Baby understand certain words and commands, i.e., *Please
give it to me?*

_____

_____

•

Does your baby repeat a word incessantly, making it a response
to every question?

_____

_____

•

Is your baby continuing to learn about the properties of objects,
i.e., crumples paper?

_____

_____

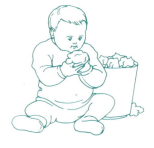

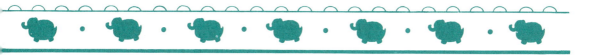

rattles a box?

_____

_____

•

listens to a clock tick?

_____

_____

•

Does your baby look for contents in a box?

_____

_____

•

Does your baby search for a hidden object if she sees it hidden?

_____

_____

•

Does your baby search in the same place for an object he has seen hidden in various locations?

_____

_____

•

Is your baby increasingly imitating behavior—i.e., rubs self with soap?

_____

_____

•

feeds others, etc.?

_____

_____

•

Has your baby begun to sense that she is an object among others?

_____

_____

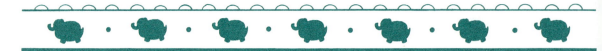

Can your baby point to body parts?

_____

_____

•

Is Baby showing moods, i.e., looks hurt, sad, happy, angry,
uncomfortable?

_____

_____

•

Is your baby indicating preferences?

_____

_____

•

Does your baby imitate gestures?

_____

_____

•

facial expressions?

_____

_____

•

sounds?

_____

_____

•

Is your baby growing aware of himself?

_____

_____

•

Does your baby react to social approval?

_____

_____

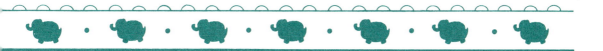

social disapproval?

_____

_____

•

Does Baby cry if another child receives attention?

_____

_____

•

Does your baby show tenderness toward a stuffed animal or doll?

_____

_____

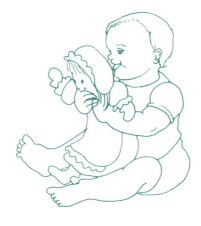

Can your baby hold a cup for drinking?

_____

_____

•

Does your baby feed herself whole meals?

_____

_____

•

Is your baby experiencing trouble sleeping?

_____

_____

THE ELEVENTH MONTH

Your baby is most likely to stand alone in the eleventh month, but her main focus during this time is "social improvement," using imitation as a tool.

Her speech is still mainly gibberish with a few intelligible sounds thrown in. She can imitate inflections, speech rhythms, and facial expressions more accurately than speech sounds. Her vocabulary includes two or three words in addition to "Dada" and "Mama."

She is establishing the meaning of the word "no," and may show guilt at any wrongdoing. Patience has always been a needed element in parenting and is especially important when your baby tests your limits. Teasing has become a fun game for her.

Your eleven-month-old may play parallel to but not with another child. It takes more months of living and learning to play with one's peers.

Fear is a normal and healthy feeling that is experienced by all of us at one time or another. Some fears are common to all growing children. Watch your infant's ability to handle fear (separation from you, et cetera), and provide the support that will enable her to cope at the various stages of her growth.

Weight_____ Height_____ Head circumference _____

Can your baby stand alone?

_____

_____

•

Can your baby stand against a support and lean over?

_____

_____

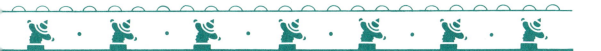

Does your baby walk holding 1 or 2 of your hands?

_____

_____

•

Does your baby climb up stairs?

_____

_____

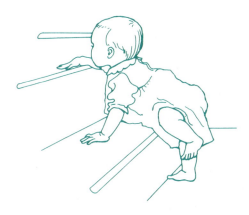

Can your baby squat and stoop?

_____

_____

•

Does your baby hold a crayon and make marks (the washable
kind, of course)?

_____

_____

•

Does your baby carry a spoon to his mouth?

_____

_____

•

Can your baby use her hands sequentially, as in self-feeding?

_____

_____

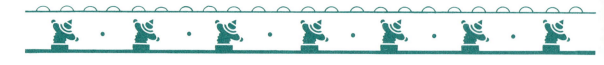

or simultaneously, i.e., squats, picks up object in one hand and holds on to support with the other hand?

_____

_____

•

Does Baby pull off his socks?

_____

•

untie his shoelaces?

_____

_____

•

help dress himself?

_____

_____

•

Is your baby's speech still gibberish, with a few intelligible sounds?

_____

_____

•

Can your baby imitate inflections, speech rhythms, and facial attitudes more accurately than speech sounds?

_____

_____

•

Does your baby mumble a word or words for long periods?

_____

_____

•

Is your baby beginning to differentiate between words?

_____

_____

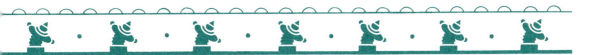

Does your baby recognize words as symbols for objects, i.e., *airplane,* points to sky?

_____

_____

•

doggie, growls?

_____

_____

•

Does your baby point at an object through glass?

_____

_____

•

Is Baby exploring container-contained relationships, i.e., fingers holes in a form board?

_____

_____

•

lifts lid from a box?

_____

_____

unwraps a cube?

_____

_____

•

pokes clapper of bell?

_____

_____

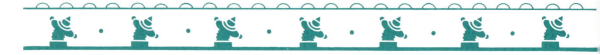

Can your baby imitate a scribble?

_____

_____

•

ringing of a bell?

_____

_____

•

Is your baby aware of her own actions and some of their
implications?

_____

_____

•

Can your baby use both hands simultaneously for different
functions?

_____

_____

•

Does Baby experiment with means to attain a goal, i.e., uses
small chair as a walker?

_____

_____

•

Is your baby associating properties with things, i.e., meows for a
kitten?

_____

_____

•

points upward when he sees a bird?

_____

_____

•

Can your baby remove and then place rings on a tower cone?

_____

_____

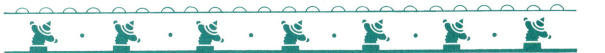

Can your baby nest a series of graduated boxes or cups?

_____

_____

•

Is Baby able to turn the pages of a cardboard book, not necessarily one at a time?

_____

_____

•

Does your baby look at a picture in a book with interest?

_____

_____

•

Is your baby reaching for the mirror images of objects?

_____

_____

•

Is your baby asserting herself among siblings (if any)?

_____

_____

•

Has your baby increased his dependence on Mother?

_____

_____

•

Is your baby obeying simple commands?

_____

_____

•

Does Baby seek approval?

_____

_____

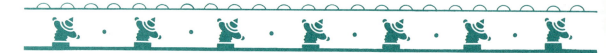

try to avoid disapproval?

_____

_____

•

Is your baby refusing forceful teaching?

_____

_____

•

Does your baby protest curtailment of play or the removal of toys?

_____

_____

•

Has Baby established the meaning of "No"?

_____

_____

•

Is your baby teasing and testing parental limits?

_____

_____

•

Does your baby imitate the movements of adults?

_____

_____

•

and the movements and play of other children?

_____

_____

•

Is your baby playing parallel to, but not with another child?

_____

_____

THE TWELFTH MONTH

During the twelfth month, you may see your baby walk by himself—a crowning achievement for him, a real delight for you. Although he still favors crawling, he'll be experimenting with his new abilities by adding maneuvers to his locomoting, e.g., stopping, waving, backing up, and carrying toys. He may climb out of his crib or playpen, so beware. As the bones in his hands firm up, he will get better at picking up and holding objects and reaching with accuracy. He also shows a preference for one hand.

At this time, your child's negativism increases, e.g., he will refuse to eat a meal, to try new foods, and so on. (In the long run, though, it is reassuring to know that infants eat as much as they need for their well-being.) He may resist napping, and even resort to temper tantrums. This can be a trying time for all of you, but patience will help.

Your baby will also go through another phase of fearing strange people and places, and reacting sharply to separations from Mother (or Father, if he is the constant caregiver). Be sure to offer reassurance and comfort when you think he needs it.

A baby's birth weight usually is tripled by the first birthday. Mealtimes should continue to be a pleasant, matter-of-fact experience for your baby and you.

For one year now you've participated in your child's physical, emotional, mental, and social growth. In the coming years, may you and he continue to recognize his achievements and share in the joys of his development.

· · · · · · 🐎 · · · · · ·

Weight_____Height_____Head circumference _____

Can your baby walk, but does she still prefer crawling?

_____

_____

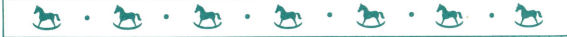

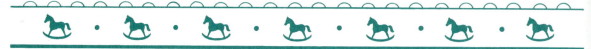

Standing, can your baby pivot his body 90 degrees?

_____

_____

•

Can Baby climb up and down stairs?

_____

_____

•

Can your baby climb out of his crib or playpen?

_____

_____

•

Is your baby making swimming movements in the bath?

_____

_____

•

Does your baby smoothly lower herself from standing to sitting?

_____

_____

•

Is your baby's thumb apposition complete?

_____

_____

•

Is your baby able to take the covers off containers?

_____

_____

•

Does your baby prefer one hand?

_____

_____

Is your baby undressing himself?

_____

_____

Is Baby producing more sounds specific to the native language of her parents?

_____

_____

•

Does your baby practice the words he knows?

_____

_____

•

Does your baby wave bye-bye?

_____

_____

•

In addition to "Mama" and "Dada," is your baby saying up to 8 words?

_____

_____

•

possibly, *no, baby, bye-bye, hi,* as well as words that imitate the sounds of objects, i.e., *bow-wow?*

_____

_____

•

Does your baby babble short sentences?

_____

_____

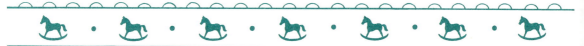

Is Baby obeying very simple word commands?

_____

_____

•

Can your baby reach accurately for something as she looks
away?

_____

•

Does your baby study the displacement of objects by rotating,
reversing, and stacking things?

_____

•

Can your baby place objects into containers and remove them,
i.e., put 3 or more small blocks into cup?

_____

_____

•

take blocks out of a box?

_____

_____

•

Does your baby unwrap toys?

_____

•

Does your baby sense herself as a being distinct from other
things and people?

_____

_____

•

Does Baby use and reach with his preferred hand?

_____

_____

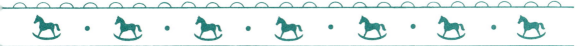

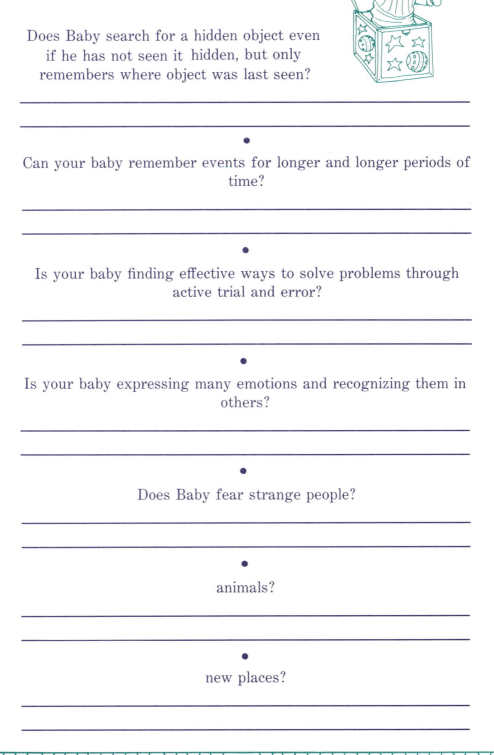

Does Baby search for a hidden object even
if he has not seen it hidden, but only
remembers where object was last seen?

_____

_____

•

Can your baby remember events for longer and longer periods of
time?

_____

_____

•

Is your baby finding effective ways to solve problems through
active trial and error?

_____

_____

•

Is your baby expressing many emotions and recognizing them in
others?

_____

_____

•

Does Baby fear strange people?

_____

_____

•

animals?

_____

_____

•

new places?

_____

_____

Is your baby reacting sharply to separation from Mother or Father?

_____

_____

•

Does your baby give affection to humans?

_____

_____

•

to objects such as toys and clothes?

_____

_____

•

Has your baby's negativism increased?

_____

_____

•

Does your baby refuse to eat a meal?

_____

_____

•

to try new foods?

_____

_____

•

to accept Mother's feeding?

_____

_____

•

Is Baby resisting napping?

_____

_____

Does your baby resort to temper tantrums?

_____

_____

•

Has your baby begun to play games with understanding?

_____

_____

•

Will Baby give up toys upon request?

_____

_____

•

Is your baby definitely preferring certain people to others?

_____

_____

•

Does your baby usually insist on self-feeding?

_____

_____

Does your baby take 3 meals a day?

_____

_____

•

hold a cup to drink?

_____

_____

use a spoon?

_____

_____

•

Does your baby actively resist sleep?

_____

_____

•

Is Baby consistently taking over an hour to fall asleep?

_____

_____

•

or does she usually fall asleep in 30 minutes?

_____

_____

•

Is your baby going to bed willingly, but wakens during the night?

_____

_____

•

Does a change of routine, overtiredness, or excitement cause Baby to be wakeful?

_____

_____

•

Is your baby taking one afternoon nap of 1 to 2½ hours daily?

_____

_____

•

Does your baby usually sleep from 12 to 15 hours per night?

_____

_____

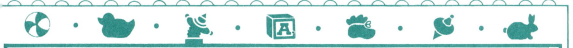

Part Three

A

PARENTING

OVERVIEW

We wish to reiterate that there is no fixed timetable for a baby's growth and development. Babies eventually pass through the same stages (with rare exceptions). Whenever you have any questions, talk to your baby's pediatrician.

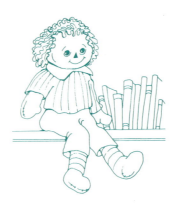

YOUR BABY'S MILESTONES
DURING THE FIRST
TWELVE MONTHS OF LIFE

A myriad of different physical, social, and emotional changes occur rapidly during this major period. From a passive, virtually helpless being who had to be fed about six times a day and night, with endlessly flailing hands and feet, your baby will have mastered seeing, hearing, grasping, reaching, fingering, sitting, crawling, creeping, standing and, in some cases, walking, running, and climbing. By her first birthday, your baby will have established trust in you, learned how to smile and laugh with you, given as well as received affection, and understood most of your simple commands.

Under your tutelage, he will have learned how to function in the world of people, space, and things. If you wish, you may specify in months when your baby mastered the milestones below:

Large-Muscle Control

Held head upright _____

Turned over _____

Crept _____

Crawled _____

Stood alone _____

Squatted _____

Sat down _____

Walked _____

Climbed up and down stairs _____

Small-Muscle Control

Held object _____

Held bottle _____

Picked up tiny objects with thumb and forefinger _____

Removed the cover from a jar ____ _____

Carried a spoon to his mouth ____ _____

Pulled _____

Pushed _____

Language Development

Cooed _____

Vocal-visual response to Mother's
smile _____

Began babbling; experimenting
with sounds _____

Recognized her name _____
_____

Vocalized pleasure or displeasure
_____

Imitated a sound or sound
sequence _____

Understood and obeyed a simple
command _____

Named several objects _____
_____

Sensory Responses

Followed a moving object with
eyes and head _____

Pulled a dangling object _____
_____

Carried an object to mouth _____
_____

Picked up a block on contact _____
_____

Reached and grasped toy with one
hand _____

Distinguished near and far
objects _____

Grasped, manipulated, mouthed an
object _____

Fear of heights _____

Mental and Cognitive Growth

Looked for hidden toys _____

Looked for toys that disappeared
_____

Imitated adult actions _____
_____

Responded to mirror image _____
_____

Discriminated parents from
others _____

Identified body parts _____

Used one hand to hold, other hand
to explore _____

Social Growth

Showed fear, disgust, anger _____
_____

Initiated play _____

Had a toy preference _____

Protected himself and his
possessions _____

Established meaning of "no" _____
_____

Helped dress herself _____

Held a cup _____

Expressed affection to humans _____
_____

Favorite games with parents _____

_____

_____

_____

Baby's favorite songs and recordings _____

_____

_____

_____

Baby's favorite playthings _____

_____

_____

_____

Describe your baby's relations with siblings (if any) and other
household members _____

_____

_____

_____

Describe how you celebrated your baby's first birthday _____

_____

_____

_____

Favorite birthday gifts _____

_____

_____

_____

A REVIEW OF THE NEWBORN'S REFLEXES
DURING THE FIRST TWELVE MONTHS OF LIFE

From the moment of birth, newborns can breathe, suck, swallow, and eliminate wastes. They can hear, smell, see shadows (six to seven inches away), and taste. However, newborns are very limited physically. Automatic reflexes beyond their control take over immediately and during the earliest months they serve a baby's needs well. Before you develop unwarranted fears because of your infant's jerky movements at loud sounds, flailing of arms and legs, and so on, it would be well for you to check out these reflexes and then see them disappear when they are no longer required for survival. As the movements come under the control of the cortex of your baby's brain (movements of the eyes, mouth, fingers, legs, and so on), and as the nervous system becomes better organized, your infant is no longer merely reacting to stimuli—intentional behavior takes over.

Reflex	If You	Then Baby's	Age When First Noticed	Age When It Disappeared	Age When It Should Disappear
Tonic Neck	place baby on back	one side of head and extended arm are posed in same direction	————	————	at 16 wks.
Plantar (toe grasp)	place finger (or pencil) under toes	toes grasp by flexing	————	————	9 to 12 mos.
Righting	put baby on abdomen on flat surface	head turns to side; baby lifts self with arms and "crawls"	————	————	this reflex persists

Reflex	If You	Then Baby's	Age When First Noticed	Age When It Disappeared	Age When It Should Disappear
Ciliary	touch an eyelid	eye will blink	————	————	persists into adulthood
Babinski	stroke sole of foot at base of digits from heel to toe (using a knitting needle)	toes grasp knitting needle and flex; toes spread; large toe sticks up	————	————	12 to 18 mos. Replaced by flex of big toe, as in adulthood
Rooting	stroke corner of mouth, moving finger toward cheek (baby must be awake)	mouth roots, head turns, tongue moves to stroking object	————	————	9 to 12 mos.
Moro (startle)	bang suddenly on side of crib or table	arms are sharply extended	————	————	4 to 6 mos.
Pupillary (blink)	shine flashlight	eyes close tightly	————	————	this reflex persists
Naso-papebral	tap bridge of nose with finger or cotton	eyes close tightly	————	————	in first few months of life
Stepping	support infant under armpits to stand	feet engage in rhythmic "walking" movements	————	————	2 to 4 mos.
Palmar (hand grasp)	press rod or finger against palm of hand	hand grasps rod or finger; baby can be lifted off table	————	————	5 to 6 mos.
Withdrawal	lightly prick soles of feet	knee and foot flex; withdrawal takes place	————	————	9 to 12 mos.

SLEEP PATTERNS
DURING THE FIRST
TWELVE MONTHS OF LIFE

During the first year, your baby will be asleep a good bit of the time. In general, sleep patterns follow a typical sequence: the younger baby sleeps lightly, a great deal, and fitfully; the older baby has fewer sleep periods, sleeps deeply and quietly for a longer period of time.

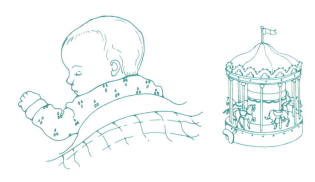

Sleeping Place

Basket or bassinet _____   Cradle _____

Crib _____   Carriage _____

In own room _____   In parents' room _____

Preparation for Sleep
(note ages)

Daytime

Special blanket _____   Music box _____

Pacifier _____   Is sung to _____

Sucks finger _____   Shades drawn _____

Sucks thumb _____   In quiet area _____

Other _____

At Night

Bath _____   Rocking _____

Patting _____   Night bottle _____

Lights out _____   Change of clothing _____

Other _____

Length of Uninterrupted Sleep

Birth–3 months _____   6–9 months _____

3–6 months _____   9–12 months _____

Number of Sleep Periods

Average estimates are 12 periods at birth and 6 periods at one year.

Birth–3 months _____   6–9 months _____

3–6 months _____   9–12 months _____

Preferred Sleep Position

Most infants assume the fetal position.

Birth–3 months _____   6–9 months _____

3–6 months _____   9–12 months _____

Signs of Fatigue

Newborns yawn; 3-month-olds slowly open and close eyelids; older
infants' movements become uncertain and slow.

Birth–3 months _____   6–9 months _____

3–6 months _____   9–12 months _____

Comments _____

_____

FORMATION OF TEETH

Your child will have a complete set of twenty temporary teeth, also called deciduous or milk teeth, by the time she is two and a half years old. There are ten teeth in each jaw: four incisors, two canines (or cuspids), and four molars. When and in what order they come in will vary from baby to baby. Although tooth-cutting is not an acute discomfort for most babies, it can cause irritability and crankiness. A hard rubber or heavy plastic teething ring affords most babies comfort while teething. Below is a listing of the average time the baby teeth erupt. Of course, they can appear a little earlier or a bit later. If there are any unusual delays, consult your baby's pediatrician.

Upper Teeth	Average Age Tooth Erupts	Your Child's Age
#1:2 Central incisors	7½–12 mos.	_____
#2:2 Lateral incisors	8–12 mos.	_____
#3:2 Canines (or cuspids)	16–22 mos.	_____
#4:2 First molars	14–20 mos.	_____
#5:2 Second molars	24–33 mos.	_____
Lower Teeth		
#5:2 Second molars	22–30 mos.	_____
#4:2 First molars	14–21 mos.	_____
#3:2 Canines (or cuspids)	16–23 mos.	_____
#2:2 Lateral incisors	8–14 mos.	_____
#1:2 Central incisors	6–10 mos.*	_____

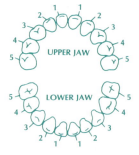

*The two lower central incisors usually are the first baby teeth to erupt. The four upper incisors ordinarily follow.

Family history of missing teeth or dental problems: _____

_____

If any, describe tooth-cutting or tooth-formation problems: _____

_____

A Birthday Greeting

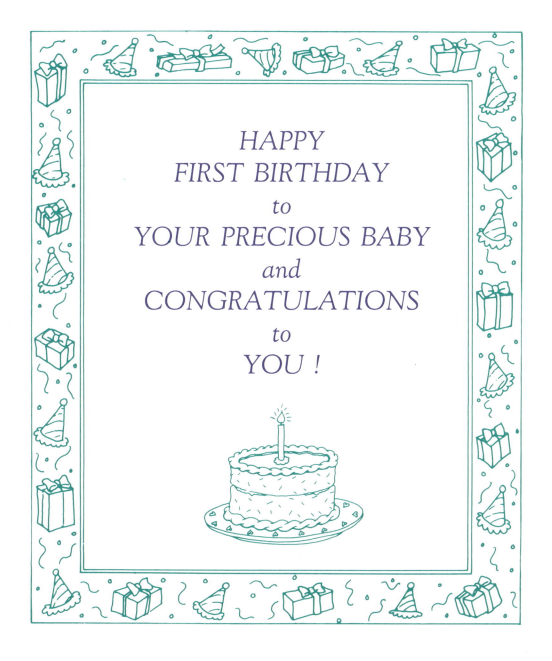

HAPPY
FIRST BIRTHDAY
to
YOUR PRECIOUS BABY
and
CONGRATULATIONS
to
YOU !

Important Terms

ALERTING: Baby shows sign of attention by interrupting his or her activity (e.g., raising the head).

ATTENDS: Baby concentrates and shows active interest in, follows, and responds to various stimuli.

BABBLES: Baby makes spontaneous, nonarticulated sounds (murmurs, coos, gurgles). Baby practices inflection and intonation as a forerunner of speech.

BIOLOGICAL PARENT: The natural parent (as distinguished from an adoptive parent).

COGNITION: The process of learning and then knowing.

CORTEX: The outer layer of gray matter covering the brain (the cerebrum and cerebellum). As it matures, the cortex gains increasing control over body actions and sensory feelings.

COUGH GAME: Takes place when the parent initiates a dry cough and the baby responds as part of an interaction process that will be played over and over again.

CRITICAL PERIOD: There is an approximate age range during which parents may expect a readiness for Baby to learn things. A critical period covers the time span most advantageous to the development of specific skills by means of encouragement.

DOWN'S SYNDROME: Formerly known as mongolism, it occurs in three births out of one thousand. It is a common cause of mental retardation due to abnormality of chromosomes. (Facial and head features are also distorted.)

KINESTHETIC: Relating to sensory stimuli; experiences with handling, grasping, pulling, feeling, and so on.

LABELING: Verbally naming everything the baby sees and does, e.g., the word *book* when the baby touches or turns the pages of a book; *down* when baby falls; *ball* when a ball is handled; and so on. This promotes language acquisition.

NASOPALPEBRAL REFLEX: Tapping the bridge of the nose of an infant causes automatic blinking of both eyes.

PERIPHERAL VISION: Vision on the outer boundaries of the eyes.

PREVERBAL COMMUNICATION: Indicates the interaction that precedes words, sentences, and language. It takes the forms of infant gestures, head turning, facial expressions, and so on which the responsive parent "reads."

PUPILLARY ACTION: The reaction of the pupils of the eyes to following or tracking an object in an infant's field of vision.

RHYTHMICITY: Implies that a child has a "built-in regulatory system", e.g., she or he will awaken at the same time every day; have a predictable fussy time; and so on.

ROOTING REFLEX: An automatic movement that appears at birth and occurs only when the infant is awake. For example, if you stimulate the cheek by finger pressure, the baby's head will turn toward the finger and the baby's mouth will open. This is often utilized by mothers to help their babies feed at the breast.

SOCIALIZATION: The process of give-and-take for establishing interpersonal relations between parents and child, child and strangers, and so on.

SPONTANEOUS REFLEXES: These are patterned movements that the newborn uses instinctively in response to stimuli from the environment. Some are fully developed at birth; others will become better organized in time; still others are transient reflexes that will undergo gradual extinction because they are needed no longer.

TRACKING: The baby's following with eyes and head an object that is in the path of his or her vision.

VOCALIZATION: Early attempts by babies from the third through the eighth months to imitate the sounds of the voices they hear in the environment.

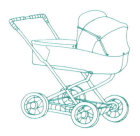

ABOUT THE AUTHOR

The Princeton Center for Infancy and Early Childhood was established by the late Frank Caplan as a self-supporting group to research and write manuscripts for books, pamphlets, and growth charts on child development for both parents and professionals. Theresa Caplan is carrying on as general editor and author at The Princeton Center for Infancy and Early Childhood.

In addition to her overall editing work through the years, Theresa Caplan was co-author with Frank Caplan of *The Power of Play, The Second Twelve Months of Life: A Kaleidoscope of Growth,* and *The Early Childhood Years: The 2- to 6-Year-Old.*

Mrs. Caplan co-founded Creative Playthings with her husband in 1945, and independently operated a successful, educational toy shop in New York City for several years. During those years, she raised their son and daughter.

Theresa Caplan is deeply concerned about the best interests of all children, particularly the youngest ones, and their parents. She and her husband have always cared about the environment of babies and toddlers, and the quality of understanding and nurturing given them by their parents and other caregivers. The Frank and Theresa Caplan Fund for Early Childhood Development and Parent Education has been established in the Office of Child Development at the University of Pittsburgh.

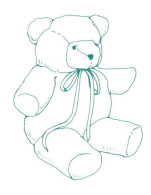